Water Fasting

Lose Weight, Cleanse Your Body, and Experience a New Level of Health

Thomas Rohmer

Disclaimer:

This guide has been created for informational and reference
purposes only. The author, publisher, and any other
affiliated parties cannot be held in any way accountable for
any personal injuries or damage allegedly resulting from the
information contained herein, or from any misuse of such
guidance. Although strict measures have been taken to
provide accurate information, the parties involved with the
creation and publication of this guide take no responsibility
for any issues that many arise from alleged discrepancies
contained herein. It is strongly recommended that you
consult a physician, personal trainer, and nutritionist prior
to commencing this or any other workout or diet plan. This
guide is not a substitute for professional personal guidance
from a qualified medical professional. If you feel pain or
discomfort at any point during practices contained herein,
cease the activity immediately and seek medical guidance.

Before You Begin:

Bonus Gift: Free Hollywood Training Program

As thanks for picking up this book, I'd love to give you a free gift exclusive to my readers!

It's a workout program designed to get you a body like the Hollywood actors you see in movies.

With this book you'll have the health and wellness side of things down pat, but to build your best body, you'll need to workout as well. And this workout will help get rid of all of the guesswork.

You'll also be the first to know when I publish new books, so sign up if you're interested in that as well!

Visit the link below to download your free workout and stay up-to-date with my latest books!

http://rohmerfitness.com/zacefronbaywatch

Table of Contents

Introduction:

We live in a world today full of problems. Obesity is at an all-time high (1). People are constantly getting sick from all of the toxins that are freely running around in their body having a party. And for most people, being overweight and on the verge of disease, seems to be something you have to deal with.

Just take some more medications and hope for the best. I say forget that approach. There are definitely some positive actions you can take to better improve your health and weight. That solution is water fasting. There's no better (or faster) way to cleanse your body of sickening toxins or to help prevent future disease than by fasting.

Water fasting will allow you to take back control of your life in multiple ways. Once you make it through a water fast, you'll come out a different person on the other side. You'll be in control, and you'll call the shots.

Your body doesn't boss you around anymore trying to get you to cave in and eat a sugary dessert. You won't feel like a helpless victim anymore when it comes to your health. Your body will finally get to shine like the clean temple that it is, instead of being a toxic waste dump.

Yes, this is possible for you to achieve, and it starts with proper education. Most people don't know about water fasting or they think the idea is crazy. They have no clue as to how powerful fasting can be. It's something you'll only truly know once you try it out and discover the benefits for yourself.

This book will tell you everything you need to know before you start your first water fast. You'll learn all of the ins and outs of what to do before your fast. How to prep yourself and your environment to ensure the best chance of success, and you'll also discover how to properly come out of a water fast so as not to disrupt your digestive system. This is a very crucial step that many people get wrong! So with that being said, let's dive in and discover the many powers and benefits that water fasting can provide you with...

Chapter 1: Take Control of Your Life with Water Fasting

Fasting isn't a new concept by any stretch of the imagination. People have been fasting for thousands of years either out of necessity, in the case of our hunter and gatherer ancestors, or for religious purposes such as Islams fasting for Ramadan or Catholics fasting during Lent.

And fasting has always been a good thing for our health and well-being. In modern times, people are sicker and ridden with cardiovascular disease than ever before. Our ancestors and people of just a few generations ago didn't experience the obesity epidemic that we're facing today.

This is interesting because nowadays we have way better advances in technology and medicine that can help treat people when they're sick. That's the thing though, if you're taking precautionary measures, you'll prevent sickness and disease from occurring a good chunk of the time. You don't need to go to the doctor to get medicine. On the other hand, if you get sick, now you need medicine or an antibiotic to cure you of your sickness.

Preventing something from happening (such as disease and sickness in this case) is much better than finding a cure to help tone down or get rid of the problem. Think for a second, what's more profitable—preventing a problem or curing a problem?

Well for example, if I sell you a fishing pole, that's it. It's a one time sell, and now you can feed yourself for the rest of your life by going out on your own and fishing. Or I can sell you the fish directly. This is the easier approach for you; you don't have to put in any extra effort trying to catch the fish yourself. And it benefits me because I can keep selling you fish and profit from it for the rest of your life.

All of this to say that companies don't care about your health—they care about your wallet. If it's more profitable to push a medicine that'll cure you of sickness rather than telling you to take matters into your own hands, then, of course, that's what they'll do. I'm here to tell you that you certainly can take control of your own health and wellness. Will it be the easiest thing you've ever done? No, but the reward will be well worth it

What is Water Fasting Anyway?

I'll explain what water fasting is in a second, but it's first important to understand the difference between water fasting and intermittent fasting. Intermittent fasting is something that has gained popularity recently, and it's not to be confused with water fasting because there are differences.

Intermittent fasting is when you periodically fast from time to time. You might for example fast for 16 hours each day, or maybe you'll fast for 24 hours 1-2 times per week. Fasting, in general, has become more widely used because of the health and weight loss benefits that it can provide.

However, a more intense version of intermittent fasting is water fasting. Water fasting is essentially the hardcore version of intermittent fasting. With water fasting, you'll first determine how long you'll want to fast for. If you're a complete beginner, this might only be 12 hours to 1 day long, and if you're more experienced, some people have even fasted for as long as 30 days (2)! During your fast, you don't consume any foods, and all that you drink is water.

The idea of water fasting is very simple in principle, but it can be quite tough if you're not used to it. The benefits are well worth it though. People experience weight loss, mental clarity, and they're able to cleanse their body of toxins all by simply taking a break from eating for a period of time. Speaking of health benefits, let's dive deeper and learn more about what all water fasting can do for you...

Chapter 2: Benefits of Water Fasting

The thing that makes water fasting so great is the many health benefits that you can experience from it. Here are some of the pluses of water fasting:

Benefit #1: Weight Loss

This is one of the main attractions of water fasting. Since you won't be eating any calories while you're water fasting, it's a great way to help you lose weight. Not only that, but it's also a good way to build up self-control so you won't be as tempted by sugary and salty foods in the future.

It's not uncommon to lose up to .5-1 pound per day when water fasting. Of course, there's much more to water fasting than simply losing weight, but check out chapter 8 for more details on how to properly use water fasting to lose weight and keep it off.

Benefit #2: Better Self-Contol

Do you ever find yourself buying food items at the grocery store that you know you shouldn't? You know things like chips, cookies, and ice cream? And then do you find yourself eating those foods at times you know you shouldn't be?

If you struggle with this like most people do, then water fasting will really be able to help you out. Too many of us lack discipline when it comes to diet and nutrition. It's so tempting to give into our cravings and desires for food.

When you're fasting though, you'll be practicing a high level of self-discipline. Forget about eating junk food, you won't be able to eat anything at all! This definitely will help to build up your willpower, and it'll allow you to get better at delaying gratification for a better reward in the future rather than constantly indulging in instant gratification. Once your fast is done, it'll be much easier to say no to certain temptations at the grocery store or to be able to avoid eating junk food when you're at a party with your friends.

Benefit #3: Get Rid of Cravings

One common symptom you might experience during your water fast is cravings. This is essentially a last-ditch effort by your body to get you to try and cave in back towards your old habits. Be strong and don't give in!

Once you're able to make it past your desire to eat junk food, you'll be in the clear. You won't randomly crave sugary foods anymore. This is a great thing because now you'll be the one in control of what you're choosing to eat, and not letting your emotions call the shots whenever they feel like it.

Seriously think of how hard it is to resist your cravings and not give into them! It takes a lot of willpower and determination that's for sure. So once you show your cravings who's boss during your water fast, they'll think twice before they try to mess with you again.

Benefit #4: Improved Cardiovascular Health

Cardiovascular disease is unfortunately at an all-time high today. Over 600,000 Americans diet each year due to cardiovascular disease (3). A lot of this has to do with the fact that most Americans don't eat a clean wholesome diet. The average American eats fast food four times per week (4).

All of these fatty foods we're consuming is clogging up our arteries and allowing plaque buildup. And over years and years of being sedentary, carrying around excess weight, and plaque buildup will catch up to us eventually.

This is where water fasting comes into play. It'll finally give your body the chance to clean itself out and start breaking down any of the plaque that's been building up inside of your arteries. It'll also help you get to a healthy bodyweight, which can help to lower your cholesterol levels and blood pressure.

Imagine waking up and being full of energy because your blood is moving around fluidly like it's supposed to! It's certainly possible and it all starts with the conscious effort to improve your health via water fasting.

Benefit #5: Increased Energy

Have you ever eaten a large meal and then felt sluggish afterward? The reason for this is because your body must process the carbs you eat into blood sugar so they can be used for energy.

Once the blood sugar from the foods you ate is used up, your energy levels will go down. This is usually when your body gets hungry again signaling that it's time for you to eat again.

The cool thing about fasting is that your body will become more efficient at using fat for energy instead of carbs. Why does this matter? Fat is digested slower than carbs are.

In order for your body to use fat for energy, it must first get processed by the liver before it can be used for energy. The process of breaking down and using fat for energy is a much more stable process than it is for carbs, which can rapidly spike and crash blood sugar levels.

This means that you'll end up with a steadier stream of energy throughout the day. Of course, it'll take a bit of time for your body to adapt because it's normally used to getting its energy from the food you eat and not your stored body fat.

Benefit #6: Better Mental Clarity

Another positive you might experience from fasting is a better focus and mental clarity. If you've ever had trouble thinking clearly, can't focus, or you've had brain fog, then fasting can help you out. This lack of mental clarity happens because of unstable blood sugar levels.

If you regularly eat a bunch of starchy carbs, then your blood sugar levels will shoot up. And as we all know what comes up must go down, meaning that your blood sugar will eventually crash. This makes your brain feel sluggish and slow.

As mentioned before with water fasting your body will become much more adept at using fat for fuel. Fat is a much more stable source of fuel than carbs are, which in turn will help you to keep your mind clear and focused.

Benefit #7: Detoxification

If you have work, school, and a family, then you're a busy person. It can be really tough to focus on your health and well being when your focus is on taking care of other priorities. Your body is busy just like you are.

It constantly has to digest food and fight off infection and sickness. When does your body have the time to properly cleanse itself? It doesn't unless of course, you fast.

When you fast, you give your body some much needed time off from constantly having to digest and process the foods that you're eating. This, in turn, will free up your body to focus on other things, such as detoxifying itself. Your body might show various detox symptoms, so be sure to check out the following chapter to learn more about that.

Don't worry though, this is a good thing because it's a sign that your body is cleaning itself from all of the toxins that have built up in your body. And of course, fewer toxins in your body means a better functioning immune function, which will allow your body to better be able to fight off disease and infection.

Additionally, you'll also feel better and have more energy. It's important to keep your body clean once the fast is over by eating a wholesome diet. It won't do you any good to cleanse yourself only to eat junk and toxify your body again once the water fast is over.

Chapter 3: Symptoms of Water Fasting

One of the main things that are going to be happening during a water fast is that your body will be detoxifying itself. If you've been consuming a lot of junk food over the years, it's built up and your body needs to release the toxins. Water fasting will finally give your body the opportunity to clean itself.

Of course, having these toxins leave the body more than likely isn't going to be a pleasant experience the first time you do a water fast. Each time you do a water fast, it will be different. Sometimes you might be full of energy even though you haven't eaten anything in 3 days. Other times you might be feeling terrible by day 3.

Going into it, don't expect every fast to be completely miserable if your first time doing it is rough. Also, don't expect every water fast to give you boundless energy either. With that being said here are some common symptoms that people experience when water fasting. ***First and foremost, make sure you consult with your doctor or physician before starting any type of water fast.***

Common Symptoms

Symptom #1: Bad Breath

This might be one of the more annoying symptoms to deal with because who likes having bad breath? However, in comparison to some of the other things you might experience, bad breath doesn't seem that bad at all. Here are a couple of reasons why this happens:

Reason #1: Salvia in the mouth

When you're regularly eating your body is producing more salvia. This salvia will help to breakdown some of the bacteria that are in your mouth. However, when you're fasting, your body will be producing less saliva in your mouth.

This means that you won't be breaking down as much of the bacteria in your mouth that causes bad breath. The best way to help cut down on bad breath while fasting is to make sure that you're getting rid of all of the food that's stuck in your mouth. So make sure that you're regularly brushing your teeth at least twice a day.

Unfortunately, this alone won't be enough to adequately get the job done. You'll also need to start flossing your teeth if you're not currently doing so. A lot of food tends to get stuck in between our teeth in places that our toothbrush can't reach.

Flossing will allow you to get to those hard-to-reach places. If you don't like using a standard string of floss, then buy a package of floss picks at the store. They're quite a bit easier to use than the regular string floss, which will make the habit easier to pick up.

Reason #2: Bacteria in the Stomach

Not only do we have bacteria in our mouths that might cause bad breath, but we also have bacteria in our stomachs that can cause this as well. Our stomachs contain digestive fluids that help to breakdown the foods we eat. Of course, when we're fasting, those fluids don't have any food to breakdown, and that can cause bad breath.

Unfortunately, there's not much you can do to prevent this. The main thing you'll want to do is avoid eating foods such as onion, garlic, or other foods that are known for giving people bad breath before you start your fast. Aside from that, there isn't much else you can do, so be prepared to possibly have to deal with a little bit of bad breath when you're doing your water fast!

Symptom #2: White Filament on Tongue

Similar to bad breath, this can be one of the more annoying but painless symptoms to have to deal with. You may notice a white film on your tongue when you're fasting. Don't freak out, there's a logical explanation as to why this is happening.

Your tongue has four different types of papallie—filiform, fungiform, circumvallate, and foliate. Filiform doesn't contain taste buds like the other three kinds of papillae do. Instead, a protein called keratin covers the surface.

When you eat food, the food you eat will rub off this layer of keratin and go down when you swallow. However, when you're fasting, you're not eating any food. Therefore, the keratin will not have anything to rub off on and will stay there. And this is what will cause you to have a white film on your tongue.

You could buy a tongue scraper or use a toothbrush to brush your tongue to cut down on this some. There's not much else you can do, and it's primarily a little nuisance that you'll have to deal with when you're completing a water fast.

Symptom #3: Headaches

Headaches are another thing you might experience when your body is detoxifying itself from a water fast. There are a couple of reasons as to why this happens. The first one is getting less water overall.

When you're doing a water fast, the only source of water you'll be getting is when drink. Normally though, you'll get your hydration not only from the liquids you drink but also the foods you eat. We tend to forget just how much water is contained in certain foods like fruits and vegetables.

Sure we might not notice it when we eat these foods, but you'll more than likely realize it when it's no longer there. So make sure that you're drinking an adequate amount of water during your water fast to ensure proper hydration and to help make up for some of the water you'll be missing out on because you're not consuming any foods.

The other reason you might experience headaches during a water fast is because of low blood sugar. When you're fasting, you won't be consuming any glucose, so your body must use stored energy for fuel. It may take some time for your body to adapt to using glucose you're providing it with from your diet to what it has stored.

This means that your brain will be supplied with less fuel than usual, which can cause a headache. Over time though, your body will get better at using its fuel stores efficiently and adapt to your fasting regime. Initially, it can be tough to deal with, but don't give up completely on fasting because headaches are a common symptom.

Symptom #4: Rashes, Bumps, Pimples, or Other Irritations on the Skin

When you're doing your water fast, you may notice that your skin looks worse for a time even though fasting is supposed to make your skin look and feel better. You might breakout in pimples or get a rash. The reason this happens is that your body is cleansing itself through the largest organ in your body—the skin.

So don't be alarmed if this happens to you. Yes, the itching can be quite annoying, but it's your body's way of cleaning itself out by pushing these toxins through your skin. Once the rashes and irritations clear up, you'll have much healthier and vibrant looking skin if you maintain a clean wholesome diet once you've completed your water fast.

Symptom #5: Cravings

If you usually eat a lot of sugary or salty foods, then you can expect to have cravings during your water fast. Some research has shown that sugar can be just as addictive if not more addictive than hardcore drugs (5)! So imagine a drug addict who's not able to get his fix for a week straight.

He's obviously going to be experiencing some withdrawal symptoms that will be tough to handle. However, if he stays strong and doesn't crack, he'll break free of his drug addiction. Think of it the same when you cut your body off completely from sugar.

Your body will rebel and fight it. It won't be able to handle it. It'll want you to cave in and eat something filled with sugar. Resist this sensation and be stronger than the craving. If you don't give in, freedom will await you on the other side, and now this craving will no longer control you.

Symptom #6: Throwing Up

This can be one of the more extreme symptoms of fasting. Always err on the side of caution. If you're violently throwing up and you feel it's best to end the fast, then, by all means, do so. You can always try again later.

Think for a second about what throwing up is. Your body is vomiting because there's something inside your body that's harming it. Your body can get rid of the harmful bacteria, substance, etc. by ejecting it from the body via vomiting.

So when you're fasting, your body is cleaning itself of toxins, and one way it might do this is by throwing up. Sometimes when you throw up, you immediately feel better. And other times you keep throwing up throughout the night and wonder if it'll ever stop.

That's why it's very important to be able to decipher the difference with this symptom. If you're violently throwing up for hours on end, then it's probably best for you to end the fast. On the other hand, if you only throw up 1-2 times and immediately feel better, then you can probably continue on with the fast. Of course, use your best judgment.

Symptom #7: Shaking

You may start to shake during your water fast as well. This symptom isn't as painful as headaches or throwing up, but it can still be quite annoying to deal with. The main reason why your body might shake during a water fast is due to hypoglycemia. Hypoglycemia is simply low blood sugar.

Normally when you eat carbs, glucose will enter into the bloodstream. Another hormone called insulin will then be released to help absorb the glucose into your cells so the glucose can then be used for energy. The leftover glucose will then get stored in the liver or muscle tissue as glycogen.

Since you'll be fasting, this means that you wouldn't have eaten anything for a while. Your body still needs energy in order to function, so the pancreas will secrete glucagon, which will help to breakdown stored glycogen into glucose so it can be used for energy.

Normally, however, your body is used to a steady supply of glucose from the foods you eat in your diet. It's not used to having to use glucagon to breakdown glycogen, so it may take your body some time to adapt to this, which would cause the shaking. Eventually, your body will adapt and get better at using stored glycogen for energy instead of always relying on glucose from your diet.

Symptom #8: Extreme Emotions

The final water fasting symptom you might experience is extreme emotions. Not only will fasting get rid of toxins in your body, but it can bring any suppressed emotions to the surface as well. Maybe in the past, you've used food as a way to cope with any stress or hard times you were going through.

Now that you're fasting, you can no longer hide behind food to cover up these emotions, and they'll get brought to the surface. This is a good thing. Fasting will allow you to get it all out there in the open.

What matters most is how you'll deal with these random emotions you might experience while you're water fasting. You don't need to try and suppress these emotions by ignoring them, go ahead and let it all out! If you feel like crying, go ahead and cry. If you want to scream and kick, then scream and kick.

Once you let all of these emotions out, you'll be that much closer to finding your inner true self. After you've let it all out, there are a couple of things you can do to calm yourself back down and return to a normal state. You can go for a long walk outside, meditate on your emotions and how it felt to let everything out, or you can take a nice warm bath. The main thing is to understand that it's ok to feel extreme emotions when fasting, let them out and fully feel them instead of trying to cage them back up.

Chapter 4: Going Next Level to Ensure Success by Setting Your Goals

What does water fasting have to do with setting your goals? Well, quite a bit as it turns out! Think about it—how many people know that they need to exercise and eat right in order to get in better shape? Everybody knows that!

So why is it that so few people are actually able to achieve better health? It all comes down to mindset. Having a strong mindset will allow you to execute what you need to do in order to be successful with water fasting.

This is why it's important to set goals that'll allow you to keep your focus and vision right where it needs to be. Sadly, when it comes to setting goals, most people either don't do it at all, or they mess it up. Only 3% of people write their goals down (6), and of that 3% how many do you think maximize its effectiveness?

Unfortunately, most people never even bother to write their goals down. They keep it in their head as a wishy-washy idea. Here's the exact step-by-step process you need to take to ensure you dominate your goals each and every time:

Step #1: The first thing you must do is write your goals down with pen and paper. This will make what you want to achieve real instead of an idea in your head.

Step #2: Next, you need to write your goals down in the present tense as if you are working towards achieving them. Your subconscious mind only recognizes the present, so write your goals down in a language your brain understands.

Step #3: Set a date for when you'll achieve your goals by. This makes it real and helps to create urgency for achieving your goal. If you don't set a date, then what good does that do you? You'll maybe achieve it one day when you get around to it? Imagine if you were getting married and you didn't set a date for when the wedding would be. How ridiculous!

Step #4: Post your goals where you can easily see them. What good is it to write your goals down, then hide them away where you'll never see them?

Put your goals right where you'll constantly see them, like the background on your desktop, or on a notecard in your wallet. Put them anywhere you can think of that will keep them at the front of your mind.

Step #5: Write your goals down every morning and night. This might seem a little tedious, but it absolutely works. Your mind is always looking for problems to solve. By writing your goals down before you go to bed, your subconscious mind will go to work, trying to figure out how it can achieve that goal. Then you'll write your goals down again first thing in the morning. This way you'll maintain that focus on accomplishing your goal throughout the entire day.

Step #6: Share your goals with other people. This can be scary, but it'll pay off once you do it. Tell your friends. Post it on social media. Don't be afraid to put yourself out there and get what it is that you truly want.

Most people are terrified that they'll look like failures and hypocrites if they tell someone and then they don't make it happen. What's worse is to not go for anything in your life and play it safe because you were too fearful of what others would think.

I learned this lesson in high school when we were voting for the class favorite. A girl said that I should vote for her, so I told her I would. Immediately after that, another girl said, "No Thomas, vote for me!" So right then and there I changed my vote trying to please everyone.

Then one of my classmates interjected and forcefully told me that I should vote for whom I wanted and stop trying to please everyone. And boy was he right. No matter what you try to do in life, there will always be critics. So go ahead and put yourself out there and get what you want!

Step #7: Have multiple goals. Don't be afraid to set more than one goal at a time. You can set as many goals as you like, and if you don't accomplish one by the set date, then pick a new date by which you'll reach it.

Step #8: Set goals other than health and wellness goals. Yes, this is a book meant to improve your health and well being, but go ahead and set goals for all areas of your life. Why settle?

Here are a few different examples of how you could write down your health-related goals:

- I complete a 5-day water fast by May 15, 2018.
- I weigh 130 pounds by June 18, 2018.
- I lose 10 pounds of bodyweight by October 30, 2018.

Notice how much more powerful these goals sound when you write them in the present tense. Imagine if you said I will weigh 130 pounds by June 18, 2018. Why not go ahead and act like you've already achieved the goal?

Of course, these types of goals are outcome goals, but they're not the only types of goals out there. There are also process goals. Process goals are the things you actually have to do in order to achieve your outcome goal. For example, here are some things you'd need to do in order to achieve a goal of completing a 5-day water fast:

- Plan a time and schedule when the water fast will happen.
- Drink at least 3 liters of water per day.
- Plan an exciting evening routine to complete during each day of your water fast.

For every 1-outcome goal that you have, you'll want to have at least 3 process goals to go along with it. Think of your outcome and process goals like a mountain. The top of the mountain is the outcome you'd like to achieve—it's where you want to get to. The rest of the mountain is the process—it's what you'll have to do in order to reach the top of the mountain.

Should You Focus More on Your Outcome or Process Goals?

When it comes to your goals, should you focus more on your process or outcome goals? This is a tricky question to answer because you need a balance between both. If you focus your attention solely on the outcome, then you'll lose sight of the process, failing to do what it takes to get the job done. On the other hand, if you only care about the process, you'll question the reason why it is you're doing what you're doing in the first place.

Therefore, focus on the outcome goal when it makes sense, and focus on your process goals when it makes sense. For example, let's say you're running low on motivation to continue on with your water fast. It's day 3 of the fast, you're feeling a few of the fasting symptoms, and all you want to do is give in.

During moments like this, it's critical that you remember the outcome goal. This will give you the motivation to continue on with the fast at times when you don't feel like it. If you only water fast for a time period that's easy, then you'll never get all of the amazing benefits that water fasting can provide. In this instance, thinking of your process goals will only remind you of all the things you still have to go through and do in order to make it to the end of the water fast.

For example, when you think to yourself, "Oh shoot I still have 5 days left of this water fast, how am I going to make it?", it's unlikely you'll get the job done. However, if you instead say to yourself, "No. I'm tired of moseying through life, and I want to get my health and energy levels in check by summer, I must achieve what I know I'm capable of, even on days when I don't feel like it. I want to be healthier than I ever have been, and nothing is going to stop me!"

Do you notice the big difference there? Doesn't remembering your outcome goals fire you up to complete the process? The reason for this is because of something called the pain/pleasure principle. It says that humans do what they do for 1 of 2 different reasons—fear of pain, or the possibility of pleasure.

Think about it. Have you ever worked at a job you hated for way longer than you should have? I know I did. I was desperate to get a job, any job for crying out loud, so I applied to a bunch of different places. The only place to call me back was a pet store, so I took the job for $8.60 an hour and went on my merry way.

The thing was I didn't enjoy that job very much at all. It wasn't because the pay was bad; it was because I enjoyed health and fitness way more than I did pets. Yet, I stayed at that job for 2 years before I quit. The reason why I didn't quit sooner was that I was afraid of what would happen:

- How would I pay rent?

- Would I be able to find another job?
- Would I be able to afford to eat?
- What would my parents think of me being unemployed?

That's what motivated me to keep going forward with a job I disliked. Not having enough money to pay for basic necessities is quite scary. However, when it comes to water fasting, there isn't going to be any foreseeable consequence for not completing your water fast. You're not going to get kicked out of your apartment, or not be able to afford other basic necessities if you don't fast.

Therefore when it comes to achieving your fitness goals, you must hone in your attention towards the possibility of pleasure. Think of how good it'll feel to be healthy and full of energy. Imagine the compliments you'll get from friends and family. This'll be what motivates you to keep moving forward, even on days when you don't think you have it in you.

How to Find Your Why

In addition to writing down your outcome and process goals, another thing you can do to motivate yourself is to find your "why." There's a reason, or multiple reasons, why you want to achieve your health and fitness goals. Getting to the core of that will fire you up. For each outcome goal that you have, ask yourself why it is that you want to achieve that goal. Try to come up with at least 30 different reasons why you want to achieve your various outcome goals. For example:

Outcome Goal: I weigh 150 pounds by June 30, 2018.

Why?

- I want my old clothes to fit me again.
- I want to be healthier.
- I want to prove to myself that I can do it.

- I want to set a good example for my family.
- I want to feel energized throughout the day.
- I want to feel confident about myself.
- I want to feel more attractive.
- I want to look good in a slim-fitting dress.

Then once you've come up with all of the ideas that you can think of, ask "why" to your original "why's" 2-3 more times—this will get you to the root of what it is you truly desire. These "why's" that you come up with will be the most powerful and motivating of all. For example:

Original why: I want to feel more attractive.

Why do I want to feel more attractive?

I want to be noticed more by guys.

Why do I want guys to notice me more?

I want to be asked out on more dates.

Why do I want to be asked out on more dates?

So I can be in a relationship.

Therefore, the core reason why you want to feel more attractive is that you want to be in a relationship. Make sure you remember that, as well as your other reasons why, when you're lacking the desire to do what you need to do.

Personally, I write all of my reasons why down on a sheet of paper. I then tape that piece of paper up on my wall right above my computer where I constantly see it. Then when I don't feel like doing something, all I have to do is look at that sheet of paper, and I will instantly be reminded why I need to work harder.

Here are some of my reasons that inspire me to be better with fitness and business:

- I don't want to go back to work at a pet shop.
- Getting made fun of for not being able to bench press 200 pounds.
- I never want to have to take orders from a boss.
- I want to be able to do what I want, when I want, with who I want.
- Getting made fun of for being skinny, saying that I would "blow away with the wind."
- I want to reach my full potential.
- I don't want to stress over finances.
- Receiving 0 offers to play college basketball.
- I didn't give it my all in basketball. I won't do the same with working out or my business.
- Getting a job making $8.60 an hour after I graduated from college.

Typing these reasons out really fires me up, and I know that it'll do the same for you! So write down your goals, your reasons why, and get to it!

Chapter 5: Transitioning into a Water Fast

Should you jump right into water fasting if you've never done it before? Well maybe. If you're the kind of person who can go from binge eating on one day to immediately not eating anything at all the following day, then sure go ahead. However, I'm willing to bet that if you attempt to do this you'll fail miserably and not be able to successfully complete your water fast.

Instead, a better idea is to transition into water fasting. I recommend spending about a month transitioning into water fasting. This may seem like a long time, but it'll be time well spent. This will give you plenty of time to gradually get used to fasting instead of trying to transition for a few days and then immediately jumping right into a 3-day water fast.

It can be tough going from eating 3 meals a day to nothing at all. There are a couple of different ways you can transition into water fasting. The first is to gradually reduce the portion sizes of your meals. So for example, if you were spending a month in the transition phase you could break things up in the following way if you're eating a standard breakfast, lunch, and dinner:

- Week 1: Reduce the size of your breakfast by 250 calories.
- Week 2: Reduce the size of your breakfast and lunch by 250 calories each.
- Week 3: Skip breakfast and reduce the size of your lunch and dinner by 250 calories each.

- Week 4: Skip breakfast and lunch and reduce the size of your dinner by 250 calories.
- Week 5: Start your water fast.

Executing a transition phase in this manner will allow your body to get used to eating fewer calories. It'll be an easier adjustment for your body to make and thus you'll be more likely to be successful with it. Each week you'll still be pushing yourself in terms of how much your fasting, and that will force your body to adapt.

The other method you can try is intermittent fasting. As mentioned earlier, intermittent fasting is simply taking a periodic break from eating. There are many different methods of intermittent fasting in existence today, but we're going to keep it simple and skip breakfast and then work our way up from there.

Here's how we'll set up our 4-week transition into water fasting using intermittent fasting if you're eating a standard breakfast, lunch, and dinner:

- Week 1: Skip breakfast and eat your normal lunch and dinner
- Week 2: Skip breakfast and reduce the size of your normal lunch by half.
- Week 3: Skip breakfast and lunch.
- Week 4: Skip breakfast and lunch and reduce the size of your normal dinner by half.
- Week 5: Start your water fast.

This transition approach is a bit more aggressive than reducing your portion sizes. You'll immediately start off by skipping breakfast. This can be tough for some people to handle. If you find this to be the case for you, try your best to tough it out or try the other method. If you've never skipped breakfast before, it can take a week or two for your body to get used to it.

Finally, you can combine both of the methods as a way to ease yourself into water fasting. Here's one way in which you could go about it if you're eating a regular breakfast, lunch, and dinner:

- Week 1: Skip breakfast and reduce the size of your lunch by 250 calories.
- Week 2: Skip breakfast and lunch.
- Week 3: Skip breakfast and lunch, and reduce the size of your dinner by 250 calories.
- Week 4: Start your water fast.

This combo approach will allow you to get started with your water fast a week sooner than either method individually. However, don't feel the need to rush things. I know that it can be exciting to get started with a water fast, and you're probably eager to see what it's like and experience the benefits it can provide you with. I strongly recommend that you take a deep breath and slow down.

It does you no good to rush into a water fast only to quit sooner than you wanted to. Of course, you can always regroup and try again later, but it can be psychologically defeating. It might ruin you to where you don't see the point in trying again. You must keep going. Water fasting is tough, but anything worthwhile is hard to achieve. Remember your why from the previous chapter and keep pushing forward when it starts to get tough (because it will get tough at some point).

What to Eat During Your Transition Period

If you're doing one of the first two transition methods, you don't have to significantly change anything in regards to how you eat for the first three weeks. During the last week, you can start to consume more liquidly-type of foods to help ease your body into a prolonged fast.

At this point, you'll only be eating a small dinner anyway, so changing up what you eat won't affect your overall calories too much. Here's a list of some good foods you can eat to help you easily move into a water fast (not a comprehensive list):

- Mashed potatoes
- Soup
- Vegetable broth
- Fruit
- Vegetables
- Smoothies

Of course, there are more foods you can eat like this, but the main premise is that you want to eat soft or liquidly foods that are easy for your body to digest. If going an entire week only eating foods like this is too much to handle, then you can eat more solid foods for 1-4 days of that last week to make it easier. I would recommend though that at least the last three days before your fast that you only consume liquid-based foods to make the start of the water fast easier.

What Should You Drink During Your Transition Phase?

If you're currently drinking a lot of other things besides water, the transition phase is a great time to wean yourself off of those drinks. By the last week of your transition phase, the only thing you should be drinking is water. You can occasionally drink sparkling water or herbal tea if they contain zero calories.

In the first three weeks of your transition phase, you'll want to slowly eliminate anything you're drinking that isn't water. So for example, if you're currently drinking soda, you could spend the first week drinking less and less soda each day until you've completely eliminated it. Then the next week, you can focus on slowing eliminating any juices you're drinking such as orange juice.

Many people mistakenly believe that juice is good for you, however, most juices are overloaded with sugar. Even if you make the juice yourself with fresh fruits, you'll still want to eliminate this from your diet because it won't be allowed during the water fast.

The main point here is that you'll want to spend about a week slowly eliminating each of the beverages that you're currently drinking. If the only thing you're drinking besides water right now is soda, then you might want to spend a couple of weeks weaning yourself off of it rather than just one week. Here's an example of how you can do that if you're drinking 16 ounces of soda per day:

- Day 1: Pour out 4 ounces of soda and dilute the soda with 4 ounces of water
- Day 2: Same as day 1
- Day 3: Pour out 8 ounces of soda and dilute the soda with 8 ounces of water
- Day 4: Same as day 3
- Day 5: Pour out 12 ounces of soda and dilute the soda with 12 ounces of water
- Day 6: Same as day 5
- Day 7: Drink only water

Of course, if you want to make things a little bit easier, you can extend this transition period out and make it longer. If you're currently drinking more than 16-20 ounces of soda per day, then you might have to extend this phase from one week to two weeks out of necessity.

Chapter 6: How to Water Fast

Now that you've completed the transition phase, you're now ready to begin the actual water fast. What you're going to be doing during your water fast is very simple—just drink water and nothing else for the most part.

However, while the premise may be simple, executing it for a prolonged period of time may not be. That's why you'll want to be sure to follow this exact step-by-step process to ensure the best chance of success possible:

Step #1: Determine How Long Your Water Fast Will Be

Before entering into a water fast, the first thing you must determine is how long you actually want to fast for. If this is your very first time doing a water fast, then start with something simple like 1-2 days. Heck, you could even do half a day if you struggled during your transition phase.

The key here is to not be too harsh on yourself. You can always do more water fasts later and build upon what you've done. Too often though, people want instant overnight results.

They might immediately jump right into a 15-day fast and fail miserably. The truth is that it's ok to build your way up to a 15-day (or longer) fast. Don't feel the need to jump right into a longer fast if you're not going to be able to complete it.

Start with 1-2 days. Get some experience under your belt, and then start increasing the length. Once you complete a one-day water fast, move onto a two-day water fast. After that move to 3 days and so on and so forth. Regardless of what you choose, make sure you know how long you want the fast to be ahead of time.

If you reach the end of your predetermined fast length and you feel like you could easily keep going, then, by all means, do so. Set a new length for how long you'd like to keep going for and make that your new target. On the other hand, if you're feeling extreme symptoms and want to stop the fast early, then do so.

You know your body better than anyone else, and just because you set a goal for a 3-day water fast doesn't mean that you have to see it through to the end. Be smart. Remember that just because you failed this time doesn't mean that you'll fail again in the future. Pick yourself up and get right back on track for the next attempt.

Step #2: Know Your Schedule

This is probably the most important step of water fasting. You're not going to be able to predict 100% of what will happen while you're water fasting, however, you'll want to be in control of as much of your schedule as possible. The point of a water fast is to be in a stress-free environment mentally and physically so you can allow your body to detox itself.

If you work a physically or mentally demanding job, then how will your body be optimized for cleansing itself? It won't be. That's why you need to clear your work schedule and stay at home where you can relax. If you have some saved up vacation time go ahead and use it so you can have a "stay-cation" and complete your water fast.

If you work a job where it's not possible to take multiple days off in a row, then start small and complete your water fast over the weekend. Getting away from people and relaxing at home may seem trivial, but it's actually critical. Think about it.

Do you really think that your coworkers care that you're doing a water fast? Not a chance. They'll eat right in front of you during their lunch break. And being surrounded by other people eating is only going to tempt you to break your fast. It's a bad idea.

Even if you work a desk job, it can still be mentally taxing and you don't want to spend your precious energy and willpower at your job when you could've saved it. Yes this means that you might have to wait a little bit longer to do your water fast, or you might have to plan things out a little bit more, but it'll be worth the extra time investment.

Step #3: Eliminate Potential Distractions

The next thing you'll want to do is think of potential distractions that might tempt you to eat while you're at your house. A great example of this is T.V. While watching T.V. a commercial break for fast food could come on, and things could be going smoothly at that point only to get completely wrecked by a silly commercial.

Again you might not think anything of a simple commercial. You might think that commercials don't affect you, but the research shows that they certainly do (7). Of course normally when you're not hungry, seeing a food commercial probably isn't that big of a deal. However, if you haven't eaten anything for a few days, then all of the sudden that ad can become very tempting.

Therefore, the best thing you can do for yourself is to watch prerecorded television if you have the capabilities to do so or not watch T.V. altogether during your fast. It's not worth risk.

Instead what you can do is watch something like Netflix or Hulu.

Once again though if you decide to watch Hulu, be very cautious because there are ads on Hulu. And even if you're watching Netflix, you must be wary. If you watch a show that has a bunch of food in it, or people eating, you'll still be tempted to eat when you shouldn't. Needless to say, watching a cooking show is a bad idea. Watching something like a documentary (nonfood related) is a good idea.

The other thing you'll want to consider is your family. You might typically eat with your family or live with other people who more than likely aren't going to be doing a water fast with you. With this being the case, you'll need to separate yourself from your family or roommates while they eat. You're not trying to be anti-social here, it's just not worth the risk of caving in at the sight and smell of food.

Seriously, these are the kinds of things that you'll need to plan for in advance to give yourself the best possible chance of succeeding. If even a small part of you thinks that feeding your own cat might cause you to crash and burn, then get someone else to feed your pet while you're doing your water fast!

Step #4: Plan Out What You'll Do During Your Water Fast

If you're going to be staying at home primarily during your water fast, then you'll need something to do that'll keep your brain preoccupied. If you don't stay busy or distracted, then guess what you're going to think about? That's right, food! And of course that's the last thing you want to think about while you're doing a water fast, so it's best practice to know ahead of time what you'll be doing throughout the day.

The best place to start is to think of some of your favorite activities or hobbies. These need to be non-strenuous hobbies, but what's something you've done before that you've gotten completely lost in? I'm talking hours and hours went by and you didn't even notice.

You forgot to eat, you even forgot to go to the bathroom you were so engrossed in this activity? This could be a different thing to different people. Whatever that activity is, that's a great idea for something you could do during your water fast.

Here are some ideas of what you can do while at home during your water fast:

- Playing video games (of course play ones that aren't too stressful!)
- Read books
- Watch a new show on Netflix
- Paint or draw
- Light exercise such as walking outside or stretching
- Meditate
- Listen to podcasts
- Listen to music

These are just some ideas to get your brain going, but you'll want to make sure you at least have a good idea of what activities you'll be doing throughout the day to keep your mind distracted.

Step #5: Have Something to Look Forward to Later in the Day

Another good way to keep your mind off of the thought of food is to have something exciting to look forward to later in the day. Come up with an evening routine that you'll go through every day during your water fast. Here's a sample evening routine you could go through:

1. Meditate and stretch: 30 minutes
2. Go outside for a walk: 30 minutes
3. Warm bath while listening to music or podcasts: 30 minutes
4. Read a book: 30 minutes

Of course, you can do whatever you like, but I recommend having a plan that lasts for at least an hour and a half to two hours. It might seem silly but think back to when you were a kid on Christmas Eve or another holiday you'd get excited about. How did you feel the night before? You were so excited that you could barely sleep! Thinking about what to eat was probably the last thing on your mind!

Step #6: Execute the Water Fast

You've done a lot of planning and preparation leading up to this point, and the extra time spent will be well worth it! You've primed yourself and your body for the best possible chance of success. Now all you have to do is abstain from eating.

I'm talking absolutely no eating at all here. No supplements, no lemons or limes, no gum, no juice, no milk, etc. The only thing you're allowed to drink is water.

This might sound boring and lame, and that's because it totally is! The idea of drinking soda or eating a sugary pastry is so much more glorious than drinking plain Jane water! Remember though that only drinking water is the entire point of the fast! This is how you'll put your body in a true state of ketosis and experience all of the amazing benefits that water fasting can provide you with. So keep going because the reward will be well worth it!

Chapter 7: How to Come Out of a Water Fast

How you come out of a water fast is the most important part of the entire water fasting process. The longer your fast was, the more critical the transition out of your water fast is. By the end of your water fast your stomach will be very soft and sensitive.

If you end your fast by eating a bunch of foods that are hard for your body to digest, it will give you digestive issues such as an upset stomach or possibly throwing up. Of course thinking about what to eat to end a fast, or how long you should spend transitioning out of a water fast is probably the last thing on your mind, but it shouldn't be. How to come out of a water fast should be the focus!

How Long Should You Take to Transition Out of a Water Fast

The amount of time you need to spend transitioning out of water fast largely comes down to how long your water fast was. If you've ever done intermittent fasting and fasted for only 12-24 hours for example, then there isn't much of a need to transition out of your fast. You can come out of your fast and eat how you like, but of course, it's still recommended that you eat healthily.

However, when it comes to water fasting, you're going to be fasting for periods of time quite a bit longer than 12-24 hours depending on your experience level. This is going to give your body much more time to cleanse itself and your stomach is going to shrink quite a bit as well.

In addition to that, your stomach will also be much more sensitive to the foods you eat when you break your fast. Here's a good timetable you can use to determine how long your transition period should be:

Length of Water Fast	Transition Period
3-4 days	1-2 days
5-6 days	2-3 days
14 days	1 week

Essentially you'll take the length of your water fast and divide it in half. That's about how long your transition out of your water fast should be. And to clarify, this is the time you're spending after your water fast is completed. For example, if you planned on doing a water fast for a week. You wouldn't water fast for 3.5 days and then begin your transition out of the water fast for the remainder of the week. You'd spend that full week doing your water fast, and then you'd spend the next 3-4 days transitioning out of that water fast.

What to Avoid Eating When Transitioning Out of a Water Fast

So what exactly should you not be eating when you're coming out of a water fast and starting to transition back into a normal way of eating? Well right off the bat, a couple of things you'll want to avoid are meats and dairy.

A lot of animal products are heavily processed, and you might normally be able to eat these foods without any problem whatsoever, but remember—you haven't eaten anything for days. Your body is in a very sensitive state right now and all of those extra chemicals and processed ingredients can give your body fits because it spent the last few days cleansing itself.

This doesn't only apply to animal products, you should stay away from any processed foods when breaking a water fast. Of course, you should stay away from processed foods as much as possible anyway, but it's especially important when breaking a fast. It's for the same reasons that you'll want to avoid animal products—they might upset your stomach after it just cleaned itself of toxins.

Imagine how you feel after getting your teeth cleaned at the dentist. Your teeth feel spotless, clean, and shiny. You likely don't want to eat anything after you go because it'll ruin that sparkly clean feeling you have! This is similar to how your body is. It just spent the past few days or weeks cleaning itself out, and it doesn't want you to ruin everything by eating junk!

Another thing you'll want to avoid is fats. Yes, not all fats are bad for you. Foods like avocados and nuts are quite good for you. In this case, though, you'll want to avoid eating any type of fat.

The reason for it is because fats are harder for your body to digest and they require more energy for your body to be able to breakdown the food and process it. This is known as the thermic effect of food, and it's a cool concept if you're interested in weight loss. This is because your body will burn calories in order to process the foods that you eat!

However, when you're coming out of a water fast, it's something you'll want to be cautious of. You don't want your body to exert more energy than it has to in order to digest and process the foods that you're eating. For this reason, you'll want to avoid eating fat and protein during your transition out of your water fast.

It might surprise you that you'll need to avoid high protein foods as well, but protein has the highest thermic effect of all three macronutrients (protein, carbs, and fat). Therefore, your body will have to work harder in order to digest protein-rich foods, and you want to keep things simple for your body.

What to Eat When Coming Out of a Water Fast

Now that you know what you shouldn't be eating during a water fast, what exactly should you eat to break your fast? One of the best things you can consume to come out of a water fast is something that contains a lot of water.

A great example of this would be something like a juice smoothie. The liquid will make it easy for your body to digest, and the fruits and vegetables that are in the smoothie will contain structured water. Structured water is water to your body can use to hydrate itself. This is different from bulk water, which has to be converted into structured water by your body in order for it to be used.

Here's a list of alkaline fruits and vegetables you can use to make juices and smoothies:

Fruits:

- Watermelons
- Mangos
- Pears
- Passion fruit
- Cantaloupe
- Grapes

Vegetables:

- Kale
- Collards
- Spinach
- Chard
- Cucumbers
- Celery

Spend at least half a day to a full day only consuming liquids such as vegetable/fruit juices and smoothies. After that, you can start to eat soups with vegetable or bone broth for another day or so. And then you can move into eating whole fruits and vegetables for the remainder of your transition period.

And that's really all there is to it. You want to mostly be eating fruits and vegetables when breaking a water fast because they contain high amounts of water, and they're easy for your body to digest. You might be ravenous and want to eat everything in sight once your fast is over, but have self-control. Your stomach will thank you many times over for going easy on it!

Chapter 8: Water Fasting for Weight Loss

One of the main reasons you might be interested in water fasting is because it can help you lose weight. Yes, it's certainly true that if you don't eat anything and you're only drinking water, you'll lose weight.

However, you won't be able to go the rest of your life without eating anything. Therefore it's important for you to understand how your body works in regards to burning fat to be able to transition out of a water fast and be able to keep the weight off for good.

Why Do We Need Energy?

Your body has a lot of different functions. It has to digest food, breath, circulate blood, etc. All of these functions require energy. So where is it that our body gets the necessary energy in order to properly upkeep itself?

Well, it comes from the foods that you eat! The food contains calories, and calories are simply a measurement of energy. So if you eat something that contains 200 calories, and I eat something that contains 300 calories, I'm essentially consuming more energy than you are.

The thing is though we must use this energy. If we don't, our bodies will store the leftover energy (i.e. it will store the leftover calories) as fat for a later use. This might seem saddening to think about.

Why can't our bodies just get rid of the excess calories we eat? Why does it have to get stored as fat? Well if our extra calories didn't get stored as fat, you and I might not be here today...

How Our Ancestors Ate vs. How We Eat in the Modern World

Back in the day, food was scarce. Our ancestors couldn't simply go to a fast food restaurant and get a burger, fries, and milkshake. They had to search for their food or hunt it down.

Unlike us, they didn't know where their next meal would come from. That's why when they did find food, like a big buffalo, for example, they would have a feast. All of those extra calories our ancestors would eat in the coming days would then get stored as energy that they could use while they searched for their next meal.

And that worked out good for our ancestors. They simply didn't store that much fat because they didn't have nearly as many opportunities to overeat as we do today. When they did overeat, it was a good thing because that stored fat would come in handy in case they weren't able to find food for a while.

In the modern world, things are quite different. We can overeat every day, heck every meal if we so desire. And we don't have to wait around looking for animals to hunt down or anything like that.

When we get hungry again, we can simply go eat another meal. This is where the problem comes in. Back in the day, you were essentially forced to fast from eating because there wasn't a refrigerator you could walk to and make a sandwich.

Nowadays, there's nothing forcing us to fast or hold us accountable. If we want to eat more, we easily can. There's hardly anything in the modern world that can stop a hungry person from eating. This is another unforeseen benefit of water fasting.

You'll be building up your willpower by fasting even though you don't have to like our ancestors did. Things like cardiovascular disease and obesity weren't nearly as common back then as it is now, and water fasting can help you get back to eating more like our ancestors did.

Where Did My Sweet Tooth Come From Anyway?

As mentioned earlier, one of the benefits of water fasting is that it can help you get rid of your cravings. If you regularly find yourself craving ice cream or cake, for example, water fasting can help rid you of those cravings. But where did they come from in the first place?

You might think that the reason why humans love sugary and salty foods so much is because companies are constantly advertising junk food everywhere you go, and that's what makes you crave the unhealthy food. In actuality, you already biologically desire these foods, and advertisers are trying to exploit this innate need.

This innate craving for sugary and salty foods may seem like a curse, but once again if it wasn't there, we might not be here today. Remember back in ancient times, food was scarce. Our ancestors had to take what they could get.

Finding a bush with some berries on it was ok, that would provide some calories, but not a lot. However, foods that are sugary (such as honey) or fatty and salty would provide us with way more calories than what we typically ate. This was a good thing because it allowed us to easily be able to consume more calories quickly and store them for later use.

When we ate sugary and salty foods it would release feel-good hormones in our brain such as dopamine and serotonin (8), which signal to us that we need to eat these foods when we can. Back then since sugary and salty foods were very hard to come by, this biological drive to eat sugar and salt was a good thing. It helped keep us alive.

Fast-forward to the present day, and the overabundance of sugary and salty foods does more harm than good for most people. Recall from earlier how some studies have shown sugar to be just as addicting as drugs!

So it's definitely something you have to watch out for. Everyone should be much more mindful of when they're going to eat junk food for this reason alone, yet sadly most people eat like there's no tomorrow.

How Does Your Body Gain or Lose Weight?

As I just mentioned, your body needs energy to maintain and sustain your life. You get energy from the foods that you eat. What is it that determines how much we can eat before we start to store food as fat?

It's called your resting metabolic rate or rmr for short. Essentially your rmr is the number of calories that you'll burn off in a given day. So for example, if you burn off 2,000 calories a day, then this means that your resting metabolic rate is 2,000 calories.

A caloric surplus is when you consume more calories than your resting metabolic rate. Using the same example, if your resting metabolic rate is 2,000 calories than if you eat more than 2,000 calories you'll be in a caloric surplus. A caloric surplus is exactly as it sounds—a surplus of calories or energy.

This is calories that your body didn't need to use, so it'll store the surplus as fat for later use. Essentially what this boils down to is this—if you eat more calories than you burn off, you'll start to gain weight. On the other side of things, there's the caloric deficit.

A caloric deficit is when you consume fewer calories than your resting metabolic rate. For example, if your rmr is 2,000 calories and you eat less than 2,000 calories, you'll be in a caloric deficit. This means that your body needs more energy than you're providing it with, and it must come up with the extra energy from somewhere.

This is when your body will usually tap into your fat stores to get the remaining energy it needs in order to continue functioning. In rare circumstances, your body will use your muscle for energy. However, this only happens if you're in a severe caloric deficit for a prolonged period of time and aren't working out at all or eating enough protein.

It doesn't happen as much as the muscle magazines selling protein powder want you to believe trust me! Yet you still might be worried because you won't be eating anything at all for days at a time. Yes, that's true, but remember that when you fast your body will naturally produce more human growth hormone (9).

This extra human growth hormone will protect your muscle from being used for energy while you're fasting. So as long as you're regularly lifting weights (when you're not water fasting of course) 2-3 times per week and eating enough protein (.8-1 gram per pound of bodyweight), you have nothing to worry about.

All the hype going around that you need to eat protein every couple of hours or else you'll lose muscle is just that—hype. All you need to know is that when you consume fewer calories than you're burning off, you're in a caloric deficit, and you'll start to lose weight. This is a great thing because being in a caloric deficit is the only way your body can lose weight!

Here's a simple breakdown of everything:

Samantha has a resting metabolic rate of 1,600 calories.

- If Samantha eats 1,600 calories a day, she's eating at maintenance, and she'll neither gain nor lose weight.

- If Samantha eats more than 1,600 calories per day, then she'll be in a caloric surplus, and she'll start to gain weight.

- If Samantha eats less than 1,600 calories per day, then she'll be in a caloric deficit, and she'll start to lose weight.

How to Determine Your Resting Metabolic Rate

So how exactly do you figure out what your resting metabolic rate is anyway? There's a very simple formula you can use to find out what it is—

Bodyweight in pounds x13= resting metabolic rate

Let's say for example that Samantha weighs 123 pounds. Here's how she would determine her resting metabolic rate:

123 x13=1,600

Boom it's that simple! Now Samantha knows that if she wants to start losing weight, she'll need to eat less than 1,600 calories. But how much less than 1,600 calories should she be eating?

Figure Out How Fast You Want to Lose Weight

Ok, now Samantha knows that she needs to eat less than 1,600 calories in order to start losing weight. How many calories should she eat though? Sure she could eat slightly under 1,600, at let's say 1,500, but that will barely be enough to get the needle moving anytime soon.

On the flip side, she could take an extreme approach when she's not water fasting and cut her daily calories in half to 800. Remember 800 calories a day would be how many calories she consumes when she's not doing a water fast. This amount of calories would have her drop weight very rapidly, however, it won't be sustainable for the long haul.

That's why I recommend striking a balance where you don't cut your calories too severely, but where you cut them down enough to make a significant difference to start losing weight.

And since there are approximately 3,500 calories in one pound of fat (10), aiming for a weekly cumulative deficit of 3,500 calories per week makes sense. And if you divide 3,500 by 7 you'll get 500. This means that you'll need to create a daily caloric deficit of 500 calories in order to lose one pound per week.

Using Samantha as an example once again:

Resting metabolic rate= 1,600

1,600-500=1,100

This means that Samantha will need to eat 1,100 calories per day in order to lose approximately 1 pound per week.

Yeah, but How Do I Apply This to Water Fasting?

Obviously, when you're water fasting you won't be eating any calories at all. This means you'll be creating a huge caloric deficit, which equates to massive weight loss. People can easily lose up to .5-1 pound or more per day when water fasting. The reason why it's still important to know your resting metabolic rate is because it'll determine how much you need to eat when you're not water fasting.

When someone starts a water fast, he'll be in a caloric deficit, and he'll start to lose weight no problem. The issue arises when that individual comes off of a water fast. What good does it do you to water fast only to go back to your normal eating habits of eating junk food?

It does you no good! You'll eventually gain all of the weight back that you lost during the water fast. However, if you know your rmr, you'll know how many calories you need to eat in order to continue losing weight even after your water fast is over.

The benefit to water fasting is that since you'll be creating a massive caloric deficit during the fast, you'll more than likely be able to eat at maintenance calories or even a surplus for a few days and still lose weight. It all depends on how much weight you want to lose per week and how often you want to do water fasts.

Don't do more water fasts in a time span than your body can handle, and don't get so eager that you try to lose all of the excess weight in one week. You didn't gain all of the weight overnight; so don't try to lose it all overnight either.

An example of this would be determining that you want to lose 3 pounds in the weeks when you water fast and 1 pound per week on the weeks that you don't water fast.

Of course the amount of time you water fast for will determine how you need to eat during the rest of the week in order to reach your goal. For instance, if you do a weekend water fast and lose 2 pounds, then this means you have the remaining 5 days to lose the additional 1 pound in order to still hit your weekly goal—

3500 calories in one pound of fat / 5 days= 700 calories

This means that you would need to eat in a caloric deficit of about 700 calories a day for the remaining 5 days of the week in order to lose that extra pound.

The Main Takeaway With Water Fasting for Weight Loss

Do diets generally work well for the majority of people that try them? No, they don't! The reason why is because people want a quick fix. They want to magically change overnight.

This causes them to take irrational measures to try and achieve their goals. They'll do things that aren't sustainable for the long haul, and they'll put themselves in a bunch of misery for as long as they can stand it. Once they can't take it anymore, they quit on their diet, binge eat, and start gaining all of the weight back.

Then once they're feeling better about themselves, they try a different diet, and the process starts itself over again. This is known as yo-yo dieting where you lose weight and gain it back, and then lose it, gain it back, etc. In order to break this vicious cycle, people need to stop viewing dieting as something miserable that you can't wait to get over with. Instead, people need to incorporate lifestyle changes.

Simply changing your vocabulary from saying, "I'm on a diet", to "I'm making lifestyle changes" will have a profound impact on you psychologically. Think about the word diet. What comes to your mind?

To me when I think of the word diet, I think about short-term change. I think about someone going on a diet, which means they'll eventually have to come off of their diet. Now think about the phrase lifestyle change. What does that mean to you?

To me, the phrase lifestyle change means a total and complete change, a new permanent way of doing things. This is how you need to approach water fasting and your weight. Obviously, you can't go on a water fast for the rest of your life, so you need to incorporate it as part of a lifestyle change.

Maybe that lifestyle change is doing a water fast once a quarter or once a month, and you consistently do that for a long time to come. Then the remainder of the time when you're not water fasting, you eat healthy and wholesome foods that help to nourish your body and supply it with the energy it needs.

Will this mean that you'll always eat healthy 100% of the time? No of course not, nobody's perfect! Imagine though if your lifestyle change was to eat healthy and clean foods 90% of the time. That's way more doable and sustainable! You'll still be able to enjoy eating delicious foods at family events and parties.

What you don't want to do is start water fasting, and then immediately go back to your old eating habits. Then once you gain the weight back, start another water fast again only to jump right back into eating junk food. This is similar to the yo-yo dieting approach I talked about earlier, and the long-term result will not be good.

Remember simply losing weight is not the goal. It does you no good to lose weight if you're only going to gain it right back. You want to lose weight and know that it's NEVER coming back. The only way you can do that is by incorporating water fasting and healthy eating as a lifestyle change that you do for a long time to come.

Chapter 9: Tips and Tricks to Make Water Fasting Easier

Without a doubt, water fasting can be very tough especially if you're not used to it. The idea of going a week without eating anything can seem quite daunting. The first thing you must remember is how incredible our body and brain is at adapting to the situation at hand.

To illustrate this point, a professor at the University of Innsbruck conducted an experiment on his assistant where he made him wear a special pair of glasses that inverted his vision (11)! Everything was upside down! At first, the assistant stumbled and struggled to do normal everyday tasks such as sitting in a chair, grabbing an object, or going up a flight of stairs.

However, after about a week, something interesting started to happen, he started to adjust! In fact, after just 10 days, everything appeared normal to him—his brain had adapted to the new environment.

Imagine that you were the researcher's subject in this experiment. It would be pretty tough at first right? You might even think to yourself, "How will I ever make it through this?" But soon enough, you'll adapt to the situation at hand and get through it.

The same is true for water fasting. There will be difficult periods you'll have to go through, but if you can stick with it, you will adjust to it, and your reward will be waiting for you on the other side. So whatever you do, don't give up!

Keep trying until you get the hang of it! If you have to stop a water fast shorter than you would've liked, remember that you can always try again later, but don't give up on it permanently! That's the only real way you'll lose. With that being said, here are some things you can do to make the fasting process a little bit easier:

Tip #1: Start Small with Intermittent Fasting

Fasting for 3-5 days or a week plus can sound very daunting. Don't feel obligated to jump right into a 3-day water fast if you don't feel comfortable doing so. If you want to dip your feet in the pool and see what water fasting is like, then start with intermittent fasting.

With intermittent fasting, you'll simply be taking a periodic break from eating. There are many different approaches to intermittent fasting in existence and if you want to learn more about them, then be sure to check out my other book on intermittent fasting.

For now though, I'll breakdown a couple popular methods. The first one involves fasting every day for 16 hours and then eating during the remaining 8 hours of the day. Here's how you could set up your eating schedule:

- Noon: Meal #1
- 4:00 p.m.: Meal #2
- 8:00 p.m.: Meal #3

Basically, once you finish your meal at 8:00, you would start your fast, and then you would end your fast the next day at noon. Feel free to adjust the time periods for when you eat however you like. As long as you follow the main premise of fasting for 16 hours each and every day, you'll be good to go.

The other method involves fasting for a 24-hour period 1-2 times per week. You can start your fast whenever you like, but when you start it, you can't eat anything for the next 24 hours. For example, let's say you ate your last meal on Wednesday at noon.

This would mean that you wouldn't be able to eat your next meal until Thursday at noon. The key to this type of fast is to sleep during the hardest part of the fast. For instance, if you find the 8-hour mark of your 24-hour fast to be the hardest, then time it to where you'll be going to bed at around the 8-hour mark of your fast.

Try out intermittent fasting for a month and see how well you adjust to it. It's a good way to prepare yourself for water fasting if you're not ready to dive right in.

Tip #2: Consume Organic Apple Cider Vinegar Before Bed

Taking 1-2 tablespoons of organic apple cider vinegar could be a big benefit to you while you're fasting. And not to worry, it won't break you out of your fast or kick you out of the fat burning state known as ketosis. Apple cider vinegar is a carboxylic acid, which means that it can increase your body's absorption of minerals.

A big problem people run into when water fasting is mineral uptake. You can lose a lot of minerals while fasting, plus even more, minerals will be flushed out if you're drinking plenty of water as you should be. So consuming the apple cider vinegar will help with mineral balance.

Additionally, it'll also help to stabilize your blood sugar levels. When your blood sugar levels are flowing up and down, you're more likely to experience cravings. And the more cravings you experience, the more tempted you'll be to want to crash and binge eat. Obviously, that's something you'll want to prevent as much as you possibly can, and organic apple cider vinegar will help you do just that.

Tip #3: Himalayan Pink Salt

In the morning, consume 8 ounces of lukewarm water with one teaspoon of Himalayan pink salt dissolved into the water. The main reason why you want the water to be lukewarm instead of cold is that lukewarm water is going to help to detoxify your body better. It also won't be as big of a "shock" to your body first thing in the morning.

The Himalayan pink salt will help to give you a full profile of minerals that you won't be consuming through your diet due to the fact that you'll be fasting. It can help to reduce your blood pressure and help you keep your electrolytes balanced.

Tip #4: Take a Cold Shower

This can be tough, but try it out and see how it makes you feel! If you can't take a full shower cold, then at the end of your warm shower, turn it cold, and stand under it for as long as you can.

Cold showers will help to reduce cortisol levels in your body and it'll help to wake you up. Not only that, but your skin and hair will feel amazing! Taking a cold shower will help to better prepare you for the day ahead, so give it a shot.

Tip #5: See a Chiropractor

Since your cleansing your body, a lot of toxins will be moving out of your body, and this can interfere with the normal flow of your nervous system. Getting an adjustment from a chiropractor during your water fast can help to keep your nervous system moving properly during your fast.

It'll allow proper neurological flow back to your tissues, and put your body in a much better position to be able to heal itself. This is by no means a requirement, but it can certainly help if you're struggling to complete the fast.

Chapter 10: Frequently Asked Questions

How much water should I drink per day?

There isn't a set amount of water you should be drinking during your water fast. The best thing you can do is listen to your body. It'll tell you when you're thirsty, so that's a sign that you need to drink more water.

It's not rocket science by any means, but it's a good way to tell if you're drinking enough water. Another indication you can use to determine if you're drinking enough water is by the color of your urine. If your urine is yellow, this is a sign you're dehydrated and you need to drink more water.

On the other hand, if your urine is clearer, then this is a good sign that you're staying fully hydrated. Finally, if you want a more specific amount that you can aim for, women should drink at least 2.5 liters of water per day, and men should drink at least 3 liters of water per day.

What kind of water should I drink?

You want to drink the cleanest water you possibly can. This means that you'll want to avoid drinking tap water because it's filled with a bunch of contaminants and chemicals to kill off bacteria and other microorganisms.

You can drink spring water, distilled water, or filtered water if you have a filtration system. These are the best options to ensure that you're getting the best water possible.

What should I drink my water out of?

You should drink your water out of glass. Plastic bottles could contain harmful chemicals such as phthalate, polycarbonate, PVC, or BPA's. Drinking your water from a glass bottle ensures that none of these chemicals will be able to leach into your water.

Remember your body will be cleansing itself during this fast, so you'll want to ensure that you're not putting any harmful chemicals in your body that could potentially interfere with the cleansing process.

Should I drink warm or cold water?

Preferably, you should drink lukewarm water for the first 2-3 hours that you're awake. This is going to help to better cleanse the body, and it'll better stimulate your stomach and liver. After that, it's really up to you.

You can drink more cold water if you prefer, or you can continue to drink lukewarm water. In the end, the temperature of your water isn't the biggest concern, but making sure you follow through with your water fast is.

How Often Should You Water Fast?

The answer to this question will vary from person to person. The longer your water fast is, the longer the break should be until your next fast. At the end of the day, there's no set limit of fasts that you can do. Go with an amount in a timeframe that you're comfortable with.

Conclusion:

Water fasting can definitely make a huge impact on your overall health and well-being. It's not the easiest process in the world, but anything worth doing is hard to complete. If you're persistent and moving forward, you'll eventually reap all of the benefits that water fasting can provide to you. The reward will be well worth it, so don't give up! Finally, if you have any questions, please email me at thomas@rohmerfitness.com and I'd be happy to help you out. Best of luck on your water fasting journey!

Sources

(1)
https://en.wikipedia.org/wiki/Obesity_in_the_United_States

(2) http://survival-
goods.com/v/9_longest_records_for_surviving_without_food/

(3) https://www.cdc.gov/heartdisease/facts.htm

(4) https://www.csmonitor.com/Business/The-Simple-
Dollar/2012/0710/Common-dollars-and-sense-Eating-less-
fast-food-does-a-body-good

(5) https://www.ncbi.nlm.nih.gov/pubmed/23719144

(6)
http://www.sciencedirect.com/science/article/pii/07495978
87900458

(7) https://www.ncbi.nlm.nih.gov/pubmed/19594263

(8) https://www.ncbi.nlm.nih.gov/pubmed/15987666

(9) https://www.ncbi.nlm.nih.gov/pmc/articles/PMC329619/

(10) https://www.mayoclinic.org/healthy-lifestyle/weight-
loss/in-depth/calories/art-20048065

(11) https://www.ncbi.nlm.nih.gov/pubmed/28521154